your job is
to be

AN ANTHOLOGY TO INSPIRE
SOUL-CONNECTION

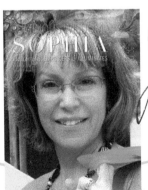

Cheers!
Susan

BY SUSAN LOWENTHAL AXELROD

Your Job is To Be: An Anthology to Inspire Soul-Connection

ISBN: 978-0-578-40595-7
First Edition - October 2018

Published by JGU Press. Printed in the USA.

Design & Layout by Carasmatic Design - www.CarasmaticDesign.com

CONTENTS

Preface..6

Introduction: Getting Soul-Connected................................8

1. Your Job is to Be..10

2. Confidence To Calm...14

3. Go There and Look Back..18

4. A Self I Could Love..22

5. Positivity is the Real Superpower.................................26

6. Windows To Your Soul...30

7. Give More Now..34

8. Words Matter..38

9. Your Confident-Life Cycle™...42

10. Middle Aged Hot Momma™...46

11. Is it OK to Be 'Hot'?..50

12. It's My Turn Now...54

13. All About Me..58

14. Do Something Terrifying..62

15. Change the Way You Think..66

16. Discovering Soul Through Super SoulPowers™.........70

17. Coming Into Your Own..74

Conclusion: Staying Soul-Connected, What Now?.........78

PREFACE

On February 15, 2017, I got a LinkedIn message that changed my life.

At first, I was skeptical ["probably bogus" "trying to sell something" "can't be real"].

Then, I stopped those negative thoughts that flooded my mind and wondered: "What If...? What if it's real, not bogus; what if it's an opportunity I've wanted and for which I've been waiting?"

This was the LinkedIn message:

SUSAN, YOU HAVE A POWERFUL MESSAGE WE FEEL MORE WOMEN NEED TO HEAR ABOUT!! You, your website and awesome message ring clear the kind of positive energy and integrated wholeness our readership audience would love to hear more about. Our editorial staff would like for you to consider becoming a contributing article writer for our brand new forthcoming 2017 publication, LUMINOUS WISDOM: Remembering Sophia.

Sibella Publications staff

Did you catch my thought transformation there? I went from What If, negative to What If, positive [What if this is bogus? To What if this is real?]. That simple thought transformation led me to research and realize: "This is a real opportunity! The kind of opportunity I've wanted!" I responded, conversed, followed-up, saw the opportunity for right-on-target marketing and I leaped!

I submitted my article and waited nervously. I thought I was a good writer, but how would an international publisher feel about my writing? "What if they hate it?" ... "What if they love it?!" Persistent thought-reframe from negative to positive got me through to this feedback: "Gentle — yet skillfully passionate art forum (dance, weaving) used in and between her words and phrasing — Clear and heartfelt message. She expressed herself clearly without being overbearing. — We feel that readers will be open and very intrigued by her words of wisdom."

They accepted my first article and I became an international writer [wow on that, by the way]. This anthology contains the 17 articles I have published in Luminous Wisdom: Sophia, the international digital publication for women [now 60,000+ global readers]. Each is filled with my heart and soul and I'm happy to share them with you.

INTRODUCTION

Getting Soul-Connected

Dear Reader,

What are the thoughts you think?

Is this a strange question? Think about it. Become aware of the thoughts that run aimlessly through your mind. Are you not showered with negativity, whether personal or activated by 'other' [people, news, world issues]? In response to this conscious or subconscious negativity, we disconnect from feelings [why would we want to be connected to something that feels bad?]. And, then, we get soul-disconnected, and we feel empty.

The soul [according to Susan] is the place of your deepest feelings, it is the place of profound love. It is the original source of personal nourishment. The soul is where Spirit lives.

What can you do about being soul-disconnected?

Find inspiration! Find positivity! Fill yourself up with love; love for others and love of SELF. With this anthology of articles, I hope to inspire you with positive thoughts that will uplift and support your best soul-connected life.

At the end of each article is a thinking question for you to contemplate. Please take some time to think, to write and then, by all means, share your thoughts with others! Don't keep them to yourself. Our world needs this kind of positive engagement. And please, especially, share them with young people! More than ever, our young people need our love and inspiration to see their own positive future.

Thank you for joining me on my own Journey. I am 100% certain that you will find some positive resonance on these pages. I fervently hope that the resonance leads you to live a more joy-filled and Confident-Life.

Wishing you all the best always,

Susan

1

YOUR JOB IS TO BE

If you are one of the privileged people in the world who can take a breath upon awakening, open your eyes and see your bedside lamp, put your feet on the floor by yourself, stand and walk to the bathroom, afford a toothbrush to start your day in good health...your job is just to be. In awareness of your blessings. In awe of the miracle you awake to each morning.

What are the stops on the journey of your life that brought you to this miraculous day? Every stop, every moment shaped this 'you.' What is good in your life today, in this moment? It stems in part from overcoming the obstacles of your past. Your obstacles, the stones over which you stumbled or even fell, became the stepping stones to this moment. Turn around, look back; see the path you trod...Unsure? Insecure? Afraid? Yet here you are in this moment, breathing still; in growing awareness...AHHH...that's why, That's why, THAT'S WHY.

How do you choose to continue your journey? Perhaps with eyes open now, knowing there will be more stones, more gates to enter, more hills to climb, more oceans to cross—on the way to Where? Where are you going? What is so important 'there'? Why not HERE. NOW. You will always be on your way somewhere. Honestly, friend, the place that you're 'going to' is just death—the ultimate place to be, the final resting—a blessing! When you get there, will you have been patient? Kind? Compassionate? Generous? Loving? Productive? None of these cost money! Already you have everything you need to be exactly 'there'. If you are aware.

I want to encourage you to see the journey as this step now, and the next; being mindfully present in this moment. Being in awareness of the beauty of this moment, in awareness of being OK with the challenges, meeting each head on knowing they make you stronger, surer and that each leads you gently along. For a moment, now, leave the doing, breathe and just be.

Become aware of your breath, then your body, then your mind, then your thoughts. What are the thoughts you choose to think? Your thoughts are 100% in your control! Take control of your thoughts through

For a moment, now, leave the doing, breathe and just be.

breathing, through quiet, nature, art, prayer, meditation, journaling, visioning, spending time with animals, children, the elderly... any of these methods will begin to bring clarity and joy to your life. Despite [or because of?] the stumbles, the obstacles, the chaos. If you are in awareness of your breath, your blessings, you will find clarity and light. This will permit focus — a magic trick to pull out of your hat, no doubt with the chaos of life. If you Desire it, then you will Focus. If you Focus on it, you will See. If you See it, you can Experience. The choice is yours, what are the thoughts you choose to think? Your job is to be.

contemplate:

CAN YOU BECOME AWARE OF YOUR
THOUGHTS AND MAKE AN EFFORT
TO TURN THEM POSITIVE?

2

CONFIDENCE
TO CALM

"Susan, how did you do it!? How did you become this new person, positive and calm all the time now?"**

These questions followed me for years after I made just one decision. A yearning thought led to a decision to change that sparked my journey of exploration into a new way of being. That thought was: "I want to feel better than this."

In my thirties and early forties...married, career, house, dog, children, volunteering, religious observance [my chaos list]...I was harried, quick-tempered and dissatisfied most of the time. I over-extended to meet the voice in my head of what I was *supposed to do*, of the person I was *supposed to be*; life wasn't fun, it was a burden. Even in therapy I felt chagrined that I was there for 'first world problems.'

It was while supporting my younger sister on her own coached journey learning manifestation, that I began to Come to Consciousness [phase 1]. I started out by just listening to her, but I grew and changed when I started hearing her. Coming to awareness of my mind was profound! I learned that I could think an intentional thought, that I could control what I thought about, and that I could implant pleasant and positive thoughts into my brain, about what I *wanted* instead of what I felt I *should* think about! Wow, what a relief. Now, dear reader, take a moment to ponder this idea, breathe. What are the thoughts you *choose*?

Feeling better, rising incrementally to a place of feeling more in control gave me confidence! It was the feeling of being out of control, of being subject to everyone else's needs/desires that made me unconfident and unbalanced — "Am I doing it right?? How do I know??" This feeling was self-imposed. It was what I saw in my mother! I thought it was my birthright, but as I changed my thoughts, I changed my actions and I grew Confident [phase 2]. Once my sister shared the affirmation 'the creator creates the creation' and I practiced and affirmed [repeatedly], my confidence increased. I found my truer self, I studied purposefulness and stayed in that space.

Feeling confident and in control is priceless. It

Feeling confident and in control is priceless.

took a period of selfishly going in, of drilling deep, of being all-about-me. My family suffered patiently while I expedited this part of the journey. I staked claim in myself [did you notice that *self* wasn't on my chaos list?]. My husband didn't like it but still walked beside me. Thank goodness. Today we are stronger than ever. Now, dear reader, take a moment to ponder this idea, breathe. Can you let go of the old and find strength in the new thoughts?

Then, something wonderful and amazing happened. I realized that there was no *'There'* to get to; there is only *Here and Now*...what others called 'being present!' I found Calm [phase 3]. Today, I am calm, living in the present, on purpose, in love with myself and others. Now, I help others go through the three phases themselves on the way to finding the impact they are intended to make in our world. What will your legacy be?

contemplate:

HOW CAN YOU COME TO CONSCIOUS AWARENESS AND STAKE CLAIM IN YOURSELF?

3

GO THERE AND LOOK BACK

B eing 'present' does not mean that you cannot imagine your future. Quite the contrary.

It is only if you are mindful of this moment — of how you feel, of what you are doing and thinking that you can imagine the future you want to create. Mostly, we are mindless of moments passing. We think there will always be another moment. Those of us who have been faced with the cruel reality of a sudden death of a loved one know this is a myth. But you don't have to have suffered a tragic loss to realize that time passes quickly. Today is already yesterday's tomorrow. Did you do, today, what you wanted to do 'tomorrow'?

When you live in a mindful way, you live in a conscious state of your existence — how do I feel right now? Am I enjoying my work, my relationship, my life? Do I feel fulfilled? If you find a positive response to your self-exploration, you know you are on the right track of life. If you are perfectly happy living in this way — great! Live! Be satisfyingly productive, move through life with intention and feel joy every day in knowing you are living 'on purpose!'

If, however, you are wondering about a different future... Go There and Look Back. Go to the future that is on your mind. Is it one year? When you graduate? Get married? When your kids are gone from the house? When you turn 50? When you retire? Your old age? On your death bed? Whenever it is, Go There and Look Back.

What does that actually mean?! How do you do that? Make some quiet time. Get comfortable, breathe. Select that point that is on your mind and focus on it. Try to picture it in exactly the way you want it to be. What does it look like? How do you feel in it? What are you doing? Write it all out, be specific and highly detailed; draw the picture if art is your thing. Journal, pray, meditate, walk, hike, run — go wherever you can breathe and think, then write.

Then, work backward in your mind from then to now. If that is your desired future, what do you need to do now to create that? What are the steps, the information, the resources? What permission do you

What can you do now to move in the direction you clearly want to go?

need — from yourself — to be in that place? What can you do now to move in the direction you clearly want to go? Be specific and write it down.

Then, when you get out of focus, you have the map to get back on track.

This is such a simple, but important exercise. Most people just worry or wish for a questionable future. When you Go There and Look Back and are clear on what you want that future to look like and be like, then you do things today consciously and even subconsciously to move you in the direction of your desired future. What if you change your mind? No problem! Life changes. Just go to the new place and look back.

contemplate:

WHAT IS THE PLACE YOU ALREADY WANT TO 'BE'?

4

A SELF I COULD LOVE

Heart palpitations... Puppy love? Or Anxiety. Shallow breathing... Exercise? Or Fear.

"What are you feeling, in this moment?" This was a question asked of me by a therapist many years ago. My answer: "What do you mean by feelings?" It took me years of therapy and 'work' to be able to break through, go in, explore, find and feel. The shellacked exterior was strong. It was glossy, beautiful to the eye, nearly perfect. "Oy, what's my problem?" I asked myself repeatedly.

I became lethargic, gained weight, felt alone. I kept it together expertly well during the day on the job. At home, I resented a lot; I yelled a lot. Then I hated myself. And gave myself more excuses to eat and not do the 'work'. I'm so busy... I don't have time for myself...What do you mean go to a gym... Sex? You're kidding, right?

I'll never forget the day I got on the scale and it tipped over 160 pounds. I 'saw myself' as weighing as much as my husband. But he worked out and ran and had lots of heavy muscles [it was just a baseless and thoughtless negative comparison]. Now, I know it was self-hate showing her ugly and sometimes mean face. During this time, my husband kept telling me something that I resisted until I had my breakthrough [AKA breakdown]: "It's not ok to be nicer to 'others' than you are to your own family." Ouch. I resisted and argued and cried False! But, it was True. And, I've never forgotten it.

Eventually, I broke. Ended up home in bed, seeing only gray in my peripheral vision; uncontrolled crying. Meds helped, family support and love. I laid in bed thinking. Is this the life I wanted to live? Is this the modeling I wanted to show our daughters? What would I tell them in this situation? Now, I know what I would tell them: "Honey, love yourself more."

Then, I rejected 'self-love' by saying it was 'selfish.' Really? Today, I know that it's the most selfless thing you can do: just love yourself more. When you give yourself permission to love yourself, you can find clarity, strength, courage, meaning and pride! [Don't you want these things for your daughter, niece, granddaughter, mentee? Why not for yourself?] When you find these things, you find Confidence—an ability to not get it right all the time, assurance that you are doing it right, that you're on track; you find Purpose that is an astonishing

The most selfless thing you can do: just love yourself more.

driver.

I found it! I started with a Values Prioritization [this took me months—contact me for a great resource], then I moved through purposeful literature and exercises [Tim Kelley's *True Purpose* book! and thank you Napoleon Hill for teaching me the power of thought!], then I learned about Affirmations from Louise Hay [thanks Sis for introducing me to Affirmations!] and started creating my own Affirmation Pix and Transformation Tips that I now share! Then, of all things, I began to figure out how to find a meditative space to ease my chaotic mind and now I write guided meditations for others. THAT was a miracle.

How? I got quiet inside. That took commitment, practice, time. Then, I went from just getting quiet to listening, to hearing, to speaking love language to my soul [the voice within]. I learned that tears are just your soul crying out to be heard; don't be afraid of them, let them come, listen, converse.

Eventually, I said goodbye to my old personality [she still visits sometimes!], and hello to a new self. A self I could love.

contemplate:

CAN YOU GIVE YOURSELF PERMISSION TO LOVE YOURSELF MORE?

5

POSITIVITY IS THE REAL SUPERPOWER

There was the day I stood in my family room yelling at my daughter and her friend...I was so 'mad' that I threw a VHS tape on the carpeted floor and broke it. What could they have been doing that 'made me' so mad?

Learning that nothing outside of me 'makes me' feel anything was one of the greatest lessons that helped me go from becoming conscious to becoming responsible.

At the start of Consciousness Bridge, I lived in superficial unawareness, wondering if there is a G-d, and imagining that I could actually control things in my life [that was Arrogance — now I know I can only control my feelings about things and my response to things].

Crossing that bridge, my eyes were opened. I found focus and clarity about who and how I wanted to be. By the end of that bridge, I learned that responsibility is what is 100% mine; responsibility is what would actually give me the control I sought. Going in, drilling deep, figuring out what I wanted was the work: What do I want? What do I want? What do I want? I thought that what I wanted was success, stuff, fame, and money; through meditation [which I now know is prayer], I realized that what I wanted was to be happy, to be calm.

The journey showed me that as I took responsibility incrementally in every area of my life—this meant stop blaming my husband, my 'birthright' [i.e. parents], my work, parenting, volunteering—anything and everything outside of myself. At the very end of the Bridge of Consciousness was the Ring of Fire around which were the blazing words 'Are you ready to accept Responsibility?' I stood before it for a long time. Burning hot, flames, hazy in the center — could I dive through into the cool, clean water on the other side? Would I burn and die? What do I want, what do I want, what do I want? I want to be happy and calm. I leaped.

I came out with a superpower! The Superpower of Positivity. I can! I am! When you take Responsibility for who you are and how you want to be, everything becomes 100% in your control! Your thoughts, words, and actions are yours [use Affirmations, Meditations,

What do I want?

Prayer to support you]. The Superpower of Positivity to be, model and teach others how reframing a negative thought into a positive one [repeatedly] can change the way you see the world [and the others see you], how taking control of your thoughts leads to feeling better all the time, how speaking the Positivity Language uplifts others, how loving yourself most offers the oxygen you need to find courage, strength, and power to be Confident, to help others.

Meditation or prayer practice offers the quiet authentic space that leads to a positive stance that jettisons you up, bursting through the water gasping that exquisite breath of air, filling your lungs with vital life-nourishment. At that moment, you become a Superhero; Positivity is your Power and you feel Confident and sure. Imagine that feeling now. Just imagine.

contemplate:

CAN YOU TAKE 100% RESPONSIBILITY FOR EVERYTHING IN YOUR LIFE?

6

WINDOWS TO
YOUR SOUL

I s your Soul suffering? Are you aware of it? If you feel unclear, or that you lack focus or direction, it's likely that you are feeling soul-disconnect.

In the first decade, we're Super Girl, hands on hips with an 'I CAN' attitude. In the second decade, something happens. A shroud of mystery around blossoming womanhood, societal expectations, hormonal infusion and for many, a slow march to an externalized proclivity. How do I look, what does s/he think of me, why am I different from others, and the sway of the multi-hundred billion beauty industry assails our every sense. In the third decade, the 'I have to' starts. Whether growing a family or a career, whether partnered or alone, there's deeply internalized pressure to get it right, get it done, do it now. I have to...

I have to... I have to.

Along the way, we become disconnected from our Soul, the strong, self-loving, spiritually-filled girl-child in us whose bright eyes see clearly, with purpose and love. By the fourth decade, you start yearning for 'more than this.' As a coach, often I hear 'I know I'm so lucky, but I feel empty inside.' Also, me...before I started my trek to a conscious existence that took my entire fourth decade. Then, I suffered for the onset of my 50th year, and now, years later, I feel free and connected.

I've learned and now teach others the tools which help you see; Windows to the Soul.

Prayer is the most obvious soul-connection; but if you pray, do you actually feel the linking with your Soul, with G-d? My own prayer-practice started with just attempting to clear my mind [heroic effort!], then moving to conquer a meditative space, then breaking through a fear-barrier of the greatest unknown [Is there a G-d?] to find prayer. Honestly, I don't 'get there' every time, but I know what it feels like now so I know where I'm heading.

Creativity is a multi-faceted gem offering your own formation, through your own senses and life experience to feel, find and connect. There are countless creative outlets you can use. You do not have to be 'an Artist' to construct the most fabulous creation

Is your Soul suffering?

of simple beauty to help you ascend.

Nature beguiles; its beauty and power can wrap you in an awe that can astonish the mind and spirit. From the simple acorn turned oak, to the colossal pounding of never-ending surf; from a cool breeze on a hot face to the phenomenon of a green leaf turning red, nature offers limitless opportunity to connect to your own Soul.

Song soothes and song stimulates. Have you felt it? Whether attending your first rock concert as a teen with the pounding base and exhilarating music making your heart rush or from a heartrending melody bringing tears to your eyes from its mournful rhythm... music can heal and help you connect more deeply than you can imagine.

To gain clarity in your life, choose any or all windows, clean them, open your eyes and look through to see your Soul, swaying, dancing, creating in joy on the other side.

contemplate:

THROUGH WHICH WINDOW CAN YOU LOOK TO FIND YOUR SOUL?

7

GIVE MORE NOW

Power. Control. Clarity. Confidence. We see it and envy it in others. How often do we feel it in ourselves?

Why is this important? As long as you have a diminished sense of self ['s/he or it holds dominion over me,'] you will feel at best unfulfilled, and at worst void inside. You may not realize it, but if you contemplate and reflect deeply, you might recognize the signs.

Over-eating, drinking, exercising, working, spending... overdoing anything is often an attempt to fill something, something that feels 'unfilled.' No matter how much you do it, you still feel empty; as if something else controls you.

There is something you can do, that every human can do, to find and feel those strengths yourself; something that is completely in your control. It's easy.

It's free. It's 100% guaranteed to work.

Give. Give of yourself to anyone, and you will find a symbiotic energy rush and calm come over you. At the moment you are helping someone else, you are outside of your own negative ego space [ego is not always negative, but it can be], your focus is on other not self, your problems diminish, endorphins release and confidence ensues. This is not theory, it is proven science. The study of Positive Psychology has brought scientific endeavor to a once-soft ideal.

In *The Giving Way to Happiness* [2015], author Jenny Santi reported "The results [of the study] demonstrated that when the volunteers placed the interests of others before their own, the generosity activated a primitive part of the brain that usually lights up in response to food or sex. Donating affects two "brain reward" systems working together: the midbrain VTA, which also is stimulated by food, sex, drugs, and money; as well as the subgenual area, which is stimulated when humans see babies and romantic partners."

Multiple juried scientific journals now exist in the area of positivity and happiness, and all agree — giving of self, giving to others improves one's own sense of self [read confidence, clarity, control] and one's own life.

Give of yourself to anyone, and you will find a symbiotic energy rush and calm come over you.

This essay excerpt in *Conversations on Philanthropy* [volume V, 2008] further shows that Giving Works: "[Seligman] and Haidt each cite experimental results showing measurable differences in the level and quality of happiness obtained from philanthropic actions versus activities that were considered "fun" (Seligman 2002, 9; Haidt 2006, 97-98, 173-174), lending empirical support to the Biblical adage that 'it is more blessed to give than to receive.'"

Apply: When was the last time you gave to someone else? How did that act make you feel? [insert your reply here]. Why? In addition to being good for the brain and the body, Giving is good for the soul.

contemplate:

WHAT CAN YOU GIVE ON YOUR WAY TO HAPPINESS?

8

WORDS MATTER

What are the words you hear coming out of your mouth... in your own head... your friends speaking? What are the words you hear in song lyrics, on tv, in the news, all around you? A lot changed for me when I began to understand that *words matter*. When I changed the words I thought/heard/used, my confidence grew exponentially; I stopped second-guessing, wondering, questioning myself.

I used to use self-deprecating words in my head and speech saying, 'I'm just kidding' until I learned that words matter. In some ways, our heart doesn't know the difference, our heart doesn't know the 'joking intention;' our heart just feels the words being spoken. Speak gentle and loving words to yourself.

Get quiet and think about the voice in your head and what that voice says to you all day every day, from the time you wake up until the time you go to sleep; and then the 'voice' you used all day still speaks in your dreams.

Make a list of the negative things that you hear in your head, that you say to yourself or that others say to you or about you. Write them on a piece of paper. Take a big black marker and cross out each negative word, one by one with commitment and deliberate intent. Then write a positive affirmation that speaks to you about yourself, your abilities, your world, your interests.

This doesn't have to be a long exercise; it can take an instant to do just one at a time. Or, you can spend time quieting your mind and getting it all down, then systematically crossing them off with that black marker and mentally replacing each with a positive antidote to the destructive decline of your heart.

I'm moved to write about this topic because of song lyrics I heard that are so vile I choose not to repeat them. I was shocked, disbelieving that these words could be put together and then published in a title, sung and given great exposure. My heart aches for the children who think that these words are acceptable to be lauded through song and commerce.

Words matter. Your words can help build up or take down; create confidence or insecurity. If you are

Your words can help build up or take down; create confidence or insecurity.

a parent, a teacher or work with young children, every word that comes out of your mouth becomes imprinted into a young soul to be internalized and held possibly through adulthood until they come back later in life — either in love, if your words were loving and praising, or with destruction if your words were critical and judging.

To acquire a newfound confidence, start using words denoting gratitude and love: 'I'm grateful for...' and 'I love...'. These small, simple words will change everything. Don't take my word for it, try a test on your own. Start on the first of the month and use them daily for 30 days. See how you feel at the start of the next month.

contemplate:

WHAT WORDS DO YOU CHOOSE TO SUPPORT YOUR BEST LIFE?

9

YOUR CONFIDENT-LIFE CYCLE™

Fears abound—fear of things unknown, fear of things past, fear of ghosts, of failure, of loss, of pain, of death, even fear of success. These fears create emotional points that get triggered repeatedly, unexpectedly throughout life. Any negative emotion or attribute — anger, sadness, anxiety, depression, loneliness, self-loathing, apathy — can be attributed to a fear. If you drill down long enough, hard enough, honestly enough, you will find the fear. If you find strength to look it in the face, usually it is not as scary as you imagined. Darkness fosters evil; when you shed light [by facing fears], darkness fades and there is dawn.

Emotional Triggers happen. Count on it; like death and taxes. As long as you are breathing, Triggers will shock you. They may be low voltage— 'not enough to cause you injury or damage,' or high voltage—'large enough to cause you injury or damage.' But, sure as the world turns, that electrical impulse will tug or yank you. Understand this fact and find a calm life that you never imagined; a formerly elusive feeling of peace about self.

This knowledge gives you power... the power to take control, to feel in charge, to be who [and how] YOU want to be. It is soul-soothing. If you know that no matter where you are in the Confident-Life Cycle©, you will always be subject to an emotional Trigger, then you can be prepared.

The Cycle includes four stages, *the 4 C's of a Confident-Life:* **1. Calm** [a place of Joy, the desired stage to spend the most time in a Confident-Life]. **2. Chaos** [no matter how much joy you may be experiencing, eventually a Trigger always gets pulled and Chaos erupts]. **3. Consciousness** [when you realize you are in Struggle; coming to conscious awareness; realizing that you are spiraling in darkness]. **4. Clarity** [committing to the 'work,' finding and using Tools that bring you calm: therapy, meditation, prayer, gratitude or forgiveness work, creativity, exercise, nature, or medication. Experiment, experiment, experiment; never stop trying to find the Tools that work to support your best Self in real-time (the tools that work for you may change over time). These Tools and commitment to Self can

Become aware of what triggers you.

help you feel that you are confidently taking charge of your life and that things are in your control].

Ultimately, the goal is NOT to cut out the Trigger stage [do not attempt the impossible], but rather to cut short the Struggle stage that stems from the Trigger. Become aware of what triggers you and starts you spiraling downward and feel what it feels like to be in struggle. Get to and through consciousness more quickly by committing to and doing the 'work' and accessing your tools. Then, consciously turn the cycle forward towards Joy, the preferred state of calm.

Feeling in control is priceless; knowing how to access that feeling is complete power. Accepting that Triggers happen, but having the Tools to manage and move through that space quickly offers you the Confident-Life for which your Soul yearns. Just keep the cycle turning.

contemplate:

DO YOU KNOW YOUR TRIGGERS, AND
CAN YOU CONSCIOUSLY WORK THROUGH
THEM TO DIAL BACK TO CALM?

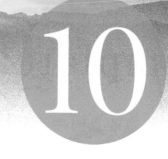

MIDDLE AGED
HOT MOMMA™

I want to be a Middle Aged Hot Momma. There, I
said it!

Where on earth did that come from? A
rightful place, to be sure. I dreaded waking up every
day to 50+. I used to slump annually around my
birthday, I think because I turned 'old' at a young
age. Responsible and a leader since age 14, even my
husband and I decided to 'just get married' at age
25 when we realized we already acted like an 'old
married couple.' We did everything right; career-
direction, married, house, dog, babies, join a synagogue,
volunteer, multitask/balance...(falter).

When I turned 47, frantically I hired a life coach
and then went into therapy to 'deal with' turning 50.
I couldn't bear it. I had just realized that 45 is actually
'middle age' and therefore I was on the downward

side of life. Anxiety and depression had taken a toll, judgment was killing me [then, I thought I was being judged by others; now, I know I was judging myself]. I even judged myself for this 'first world problem' knowing how many others suffered just for food, or through illness or loss — what was my problem?

Good fortune had my primary doctor tell me that if I wanted to get off medication, I should go to the gym [I did]. Then, more good fortune landed my daughter moving home after college with a desire to become a personal trainer. My desire to have us connect personally in adult fun resulted in working together to get me from zero to a half marathon. That 13.1 day was a defining moment for me. From then to now I have found calm in my age, my place, my journey, my purpose. I am a Middle Aged Hot Momma! You?

Before you let the self-doubt demons shout denial, hear me out. A Middle Aged Hot Momma is connected to self-energy, comfortable in her own skin, has a prosperous mindset and a healthy lifestyle. Now, can you see yourself this way?

Break through negative self-speak to a better self-image, improve your self-talk! Learn about the concept that *Thoughts Are Things* [Prentice Mulford], things you can control if you have a desire to feel better. Controlled thoughts can be transformed from negative to positive to superlative. Then, turn your attention

Break through negative self-speak to a better self-image.

to your body. Not about how it looks, but rather how it feels. Do you feel fit and strong? Through desire and commitment to living a stronger, fitter life, you can motivate yourself to get off the couch, walk an extra mile, or lift a kettlebell. Next, visit with your soul. Explore Self through journaling; then have soul-filled conversations with people you love and trust, ask deep questions, share freely and listen openly.

If you desire a self-fulfilled and purposeful second half of life, consider joining the club of women consciously moving confidently through life. It's 100% in your control if you choose.

contemplate:

WHAT GOOD DO YOU SEE IN YOUR SECOND HALF?

11

IS IT OK TO
BE 'HOT?'

R eally? At our age, we're asking if it's okay to be Hot? In light of newfound awareness through #MeToo and #TimesUp, should I be more prudent than to create a brand using the word 'Hot?' First, I pray there is a transformed consciousness and transformation of behavior about how to engage with girls and women at this extraordinary time in history. I ache for the girls of the past who were abused, for the women of the past who were preyed upon and tortured; for the people of the past who allowed it to be so. As a lightworker, I work to shed light on those ills and as a person of faith, I must leave those souls in the place they found rest.

Today, my goal as an influencer is to transform the meaning of 'Hot' from sexy to Confident. Realistic? I don't know, but a worthy endeavor. Even the sexiest among us often don't see themselves that way; read interviews with models and movie stars to know of their inner 'truth' and personal insecurities. Ironically, it is only the women who have the highest level of self-confidence and self-love who really feel sexy in their own skin, stemming from an internal sense of self, not from an external slinky gown. If older women can get/feel/share this concept, younger women will learn/absorb/benefit!

Let's get to the sex part of 'Hot:' By middle age, most of us have likely had some pretty sexy and sex-filled years. I have a growing awareness of middle-aged women being done with sex (yes, I went there). This is a total disconnect from what men want and what women say they want. Whether you're in a healthy partnership or wanting companionship, it seems like sex is a desired thing. I am not a sex expert nor equipped to give a professional opinion on this topic. I could share anecdotally my own experience—I won't, however, to spare my daughter's mortification! But, I can say that through my coaching practice many middle-aged women have talked to me about dryness, pain, taking too long, lack of desire, fatigue, etc. The topic comes up in coaching conversations about what do you want in your life, overall wellness and the 'life I want to live.'

My goal is for you to feel comfortable in your own skin and confident with your body and to be intimate

My goal is for you to feel comfortable in your own skin.

if this is your desire. For sure, we will not be comfortable being intimate if we're not comfortable in our own skin, no? And, back to HOTNESS, sex isn't even in the equation! I had to bring it up in order to get it out of your mind, but it doesn't go Sex to Sexy, it goes Confident to Sexy to Sex! Get it? You get to decide about the physical outlet for your newfound confident sexy self! Is it ok to be 'Hot?' You bet it is!

contemplate:

HOW CAN YOU GET COMFORTABLE IN YOUR OWN SKIN?

12

IT'S MY TURN NOW

I t's my turn now.

"What do those words even mean? I know what each individual word means, but I'm having trouble processing what the phrase means to me." These are commonly heard responses when I ask women clients to say the words out loud to themselves.

Starting as young girls, we observe and absorb family, societal and generational expectations that we become nurturers. Take care of your little brother, help out around the house, be a helper to your mother, call your grandparents, go help the neighbor — most women today would recognize these phrases and doubtless more. "It's just what I do" they tell me. Tending to everyone's every need is a wonderful characteristic; being the Superhero Kool-aid Mom is an aspiration for many. And, for those who do not have children, by choice or by G-d, there is still a going-out-of oneself. The Nurture Syndrome manifests in other ways — as the person at work who 'has the time' and does it all, or the volunteer at church who never says no. But virtually most women feel they fall short.

Stay-at-home moms lose themselves. External career-path moms live with incessant guilt. Each thinks the other has it better: "I wish I could make the cookies and bring them in for the classroom activity." "I wish I could dress up in a suit and go to a business luncheon with other adults."

Along the way, while nurturing others — doing more, giving more, tending more — you begin to forego the things you used to love. Playing softball, hiking or running, spending weekends baking, going out with friends shopping, even just long phone calls with your sister/friend talking about life. 'Self' gets hidden or buried while 'other' takes precedence in your mind and in your life. It's slow, insidious, and by the time a decade passes, you're lost in the rote behavior. You move this way on autopilot, further depleting the self for another decade or more.

Then, something happens that wakes you up. Perhaps it's empty-nesting, turning age 50, losing your best-friend mom, or an illness. Suddenly, you become aware of your lost self. "I used to love to read for hours on end..." "I remember how praying for 20 minutes

You become aware of your lost self.

every morning grounded me..." "When was the last time I wrote a letter to my aunt? I used to tell her everything."

What would happen if you said "It's my turn now" and honored those words? Does it mean you are forsaking everyone else or your responsibilities? No, of course not. We're women! It's impossible to not care for and about others. But in honoring those words, we'll take back our self-power. In so doing, we'll be more impactful, more persuasive, more productive — the world will win when we take back our self-power. Putting the oxygen mask on yourself first shores you up to help others as you are meant to do.

contemplate:

WHAT DID YOU LOVE TO DO THAT YOU'VE MISSED?

13

ALL ABOUT ME

"I rock. I love and revere the impact I make." I stand by this statement and I apologize for nothing. Why should I apologize? I think deeply, I work hard, I am committed to using my skills, talents, and heart to create a greater good in our world while I'm in it. And, most of all, I want to role model to younger women the value of seeing one's own worth and feeling self-confidence *which allows greater impact.*

As women, we nurture. Whether it is innate, ordained, encouraged or imposed, nurturing others, lifting up or helping others is what we do. While this is a wonderful characteristic, and promulgated by religion, society and our parents as 'worthy,' it can also lead down a negative rabbit-hole to low esteem or self-subjugation. Often, we lift up others at the expense of ourselves.

In their book, *How Women Rise*, Sally Helgesen, and Marshall Goldsmith expound on this important topic in their chapter about the very first Habit [of twelve habits holding you back from your next raise, promotion, or job]: *Reluctance to Claim Your Achievements*. In a section titled 'The Art of Self-Promotion,' they say: "Speaking up about what you contribute and detailing why you're qualified does not make you self-centered or self-serving. It sends a signal that you're ready to rise." And this: "If you don't find a way to speak about the value of what you're doing, you send a message that you don't put much value on it. And if you don't value it, why should anyone else?"

Whether you are a mom volunteering as a Girl Scout leader, a corporate VP, or a solopreneur coaching others to live their best life, it is vital to take an intentional stroll around the 'all about me' block. NOT arrogant, NOT egotistical, rather it is akin to putting on the oxygen mask first. Self-love — allowing it to be all about you for a while — is an act that will sanction confidence, and as a result, more impact, more uplifting of others and greater results. What is more nurturing than that?

I arrive at the same place we started: "as women, we nurture." But I arrive there from a position of self-strength, not self-subjugation; lovingly living our own best lives and by example and through our work, helping others do the same. Make this year all about

Make this year all about you.

you. Think deeply, figure out what matters to you and where you choose to focus your best efforts. Make your own choice to commit and act accordingly; that's you in full control. Enjoy the feeling.

contemplate:

CAN YOU GET COMFORTABLE
WITH ALLOWING IT TO BE ALL
ABOUT YOU FOR A TIME?

14

DO SOMETHING TERRIFYING

When was the last time you did something terrifying? Terrifying in a good way, as in "Oh my gosh, I'm really doing this?!" Can you think of anything in the last few or several years? Or was it when you were younger? Even for a person who, as an adult plays it safe and does not like risk, there was likely a time in your life that you did something like throw yourself rolling down a hill with other children, fearful heart-beating excitedly, laughing all the way down or danced wildly uninhibited at one Rave. Can you remember that feeling?

Often, as a momma-bear or momma-worker [someone who nurtures everyone else at work], we don't feel we have the luxury of doing something exhilarating for ourselves; nay, we create and give those opportunities to others. If you go through the day tending to everything that 'has to' get done — from rising to retiring — consider doing something terrifying — in the good way. If you feel like a rote robot most days, I say: Momma, it's Your Turn Now.

Feeling terrified to do something new or hard is a great activity for you to consider if you are in the second half of your life [which actually starts around age 43!]. Feeling terrified — in the good way — generates energy and excitement. It feels like enthusiasm bubbling over every day, it creates a secret-in-you that no one else can guess. It even creates endorphins. Endorphins create the hormone-high you get when you exercise. Yes, exercise, you know, when you run that 10k race or hit the court for a set of doubles? OK, I know that is laughable. Who has time to train for and run a 10k?

Some women get the exhilaration, the endorphins from sex — perhaps a more frequent activity earlier in your life; but some middle-aged or older women [many, most?] do not. If you are inspired, I encourage you to try this method of creating excited energy in your life! Have fun [be safe]! As an aside, when you bring excited endorphin-filled energy back in your life, your sex-life can benefit because you feel Hot [confident] and younger!

What are ways you can do something terrifying — in the good way? I'm doing it by writing a book. I

What if I succeed?

have long had a book in me, but only recently gave myself permission [time, money, and energy] to go for it. It's terrifyingly exhilarating. What if I succeed? What if I fail? It's risk beyond my norm; I'm going for it. Now, I wake up every day with a new energy, a new purpose; one that is outside of my 30+ year career. You don't have to write a book, but maybe you set a big activity, travel, weight or public speaking goal, commit to it heart-and-soul and go for it? Do that thing now! Do that thing that you've long wanted and long-suppressed. Don't wait another moment. Feel the energy? It's Your Turn Now.

contemplate:

WHAT TERRIFYING THING WOULD ALSO BE EXHILARATING TO YOU?

15

CHANGE THE
WAY YOU THINK

....

"What do they need?"

Is this a recurring thought for you about your children, your parents, your work team or volunteer group? For most women, this thought begins to crop up in the late twenties and it continues unabated for the next twenty years. For those forced to become 'parents' early—e.g. for siblings of alcoholic parents—this thought starts even earlier in life.

"What do they need...today, this week, this school year, this quarter?" As women we nurture and often we enable. How many women do you know who are still cooking for and serving their 20-something children living at home? Or, bringing work home nights and weekends to cover for inept or inexperienced people? Or, who work doubles or do overtime at work OR home while also supporting aging parents? You get my point.

Take a breath, we all do the best we can! Take another cleansing breath and wonder [get curious]: could it be different? Is it time? Is now the time to start thinking differently? Even if people are still currently dependent on you, could there be a crack in that 'I have to' armor you've worn for all these years? Is it possible that others might be able to, may even want to *support you* to have a fulfilling and purposeful second half of life, for you to break out of the box that started getting built around you decades ago?

It's not a bad thing to help others, to *want* to nurture, love, support, even enable. It's just that after decades of living this way, it leads to loss of *self* [asking yourself 'who is that?' when you look in the mirror, wondering 'What happened to me?'].

The changing picture of self starts with a changing mindset, with getting control of your mind, of your thoughts. Instead of 'What do they need,' imagine thoughts like: 'Is it my turn now?' 'What would happen if...[I took a night a week for my hobby/passion]?' 'What would happen if I went away to a conference on a 'soft' topic that will enhance my leadership for my team?' 'Will my loved ones/team be ok?'

The changing picture of self starts with a changing mindset.

Changing your mindset from *others* to *self* takes time, commitment, but mostly desire. You must want to begin to change the way you see yourself in order for others to change what they see/experience in you. Consider it with love for yourself, and for your second half of life. And, as great role modeling for everyone, especially for the girls and younger women in your life. Is it possible for them to do it differently? Do they have to 'lose themselves' along their life's journey? Or, if we show them at a younger age how to connect, love themselves, and collaborate and partner more effectively with others, might they come into their mature years in joy and strength, on purpose and fulfilled in a way that we only wish we were today, at this life stage?

contemplate:

IT'S MY TURN NOW [AND FOR
THE SECOND HALF OF MY LIFE],
WHAT DO I NEED RIGHT NOW?

16

DISCOVERING SOUL THROUGH SUPER SOULPOWERS©

A re you soul-connected? Or, soul-disconnected?

Like a diamond buried deep in the earth, your soul waits to be discovered and extracted, the rock layers chipped away, the gem within, cut and polished to a gleaming treasure, its facets glittering in the light with each turn. Your soul is multifaceted and so valuable; invaluable, really. Each surface smooth and gleaming, light rays shining through. And unlimited! Our soul has personas made up of every experience we've had, every person who has touched our lives, every thought that has been 'thunk' and every feeling that has been felt. Your soul is on-point, on-purpose and on-call; there for the asking, to support your best life at any minute. BUT, as with a diamond that must be mined, so too, must our soul be painstakingly uncovered.

Doing this takes superhero power! [You know I'm right.] To fight against complacency, lethargy, apathy, overwhelm, anger, sadness and the hardest fight of all, fear. When you are suffering, sometimes it takes heroic effort to rise above it all. To help you get there, to uncover your soul's yearning to feel peace, your soul's desire to 'come out,' imagine yourself as that superhero, with superpowers to help you get connected.

I call them Super SoulPowers™. The first one is Love [doesn't everything start with love?], and the others emanate out from there. There is a priority order, each one builds from the kernel of the first, mightiest power:

Super SoulPower #1: Love. Love for yourself, your best efforts and intentions, and for the failures, too. And, love of others, unconditional love; but not the kind that deprecates or subjugates yourself. When you love yourself, you can live in

Super SoulPower #2: Truth. Get quiet, go in and deep; listen. What do you hear? Use your breath to get focused and get even quieter. Listen again, what do you hear now? Your soul will speak your Truth. When you live in Truth, you can find

Super SoulPower #3: Forgiveness. Not forgiveness of others, though that is a nice thing to do; forgiveness

Your soul is multifaceted and so valuable.

of yourself. Forgiving yourself your failures, your ineptitude and any other self-hating attributes you heap on your own head. When you've forgiven yourself your frailty, you can feel

Super SoulPower #4: Gratitude. Gratitude for love, for quiet, for truth, for all that you are, and for all that you have. Gratitude to self, to self-acclaim, and of course, gratitude to the greatest universal source, for life. When you feel Gratitude, then you can achieve

Super SoulPower #5: Positivity. This tangible scientifically-proven power can transform your thoughts and your being. It offers the final connection to joy. Once you can feel joy, you can find calm.

And, when you are calm — no matter the circumstances of your life, your soul shines, you are soul-connected.

contemplate:

HOW CAN YOU USE THE SUPER SOULPOWERS™ TO GET YOU THROUGH A DIFFICULT TIME?

17

COMING INTO
MY OWN

Dear Younger Self: Appreciate the sun and the moon, the tides and the sand, the rain, and the wind. And your breath. Appreciate your breath more. These are the markers of life. Material things are nice, they are not unimportant. But in the end, when things get so hard that you think you cannot bear it, there is one thing that you can still rely on — the earth will rotate, dawn will arrive. So, make more time to sit in nature and breathe, just breathe. Feel your breath connecting to the essence of the earth, the tone of the tides, or the majesty of the mountains.

Please know that it is ok to believe in G-d as the universal source of all that is. But, know, too that it is free will and choice that is your connection to Self. This connection will support you throughout the perilous journey that is one's life.

From the moment you become a sentient human, there is a question that you begin to ask yourself that never goes away: "Am I Ok?" It becomes gradient, taking on mass proportions in later years. The "Am I going to fall?" thought you might have from learning to walk turns into "Am I going to fail?" about, well, everything throughout the stages of life. There is a glory-time when girls hit a power-stride at about age 6 or 7; "I CAN" exudes, "I WILL" comes forth, "I AM" lasts for another few years. Take a moment now to breathe, reflect and try to connect to your inner 8-year-old-she's in there; what do you remember about her? Give your Self over to her fearlessness for a moment. Breathe.

What happened to that girl? Many things, each one acting like a relentless sledgehammer pounding her down: advertising, puberty, Mean Girls, boys, lack of strong women role models, self-questioning, Good-Girl syndrome. She was gloriously internal for her developing earliest years, so many thoughts within; everything was a wonder. But exposure to life brought her outward, to the external self that would be thrashed about for decades, often ending up like a wet rag on the floor. Hyperbole? No. Reality.

To that self I want to say: Honeypie, know, just know that there will be a time that you come into your own. If not sooner perhaps, then when you reach your late-middle age years, there is a freedom the likes of which you cannot imagine now. There appears to be

Appreciate your breath more.

some magic about aging into this stage if you allow it. Perhaps it's from the self-knowledge of: "DID IT" [often followed by "Don't know how well, but at least it's done"]. Whether it's the launch of your children or for those with no children, the launch from later-career success, turning 50 can bring the beginning of an awareness that grows and grows. 60 [as I observe] can bring the liberation of breaking through. There is that last filmy layer, diaphanously fluttering in front of you, inviting you to step through, to see your old friends again! Hello! There in front of you in clear opulent vision are the sun, the moon, the trees, mountains, and tides. Wow, breathe that in! And, breathe again quietly.

Coming into my own. Can it happen sooner? Yes! It can! If you want it; if you figure out what that means to you. If you give yourself permission, and if you allow it. What does it mean to you? Connect back to your source, not to the material things, not to the success that others project. Go in, go deep. Come into your own, now.

contemplate:

WHAT DOES IT MEAN TO YOU TO COME INTO YOUR OWN?

CONCLUSION

Staying Soul-Connected, What Now?

Dear Friend,

I started the introduction of this book with "Dear Reader."

Now, after our journey together through these pages, I call you Friend,

So, Friend, what now? Now that you have taken time for yourself, time to read, reflect, write and share with others these positive ideas, messages and thoughts, how will you hold onto them, keep them integrated into your life and apply them daily? AKA: how will you stay soul-connected?

How will you live your life, now, this minute, this hour, this day [on the way to the rest of your life]? Will you choose to live in a mindful soul-connected way? Or fall mindlessly back into rote or negative thinking, forgetting the power of choosing your thoughts?

Are you familiar with this quote from Louise Hay [it changed my life]:

> "How you start your day
> is often how you live your life."

In other words, how you start your day leads to how you continue your day, how you go on with the rest of the day and how you end your day. What are the feelings you have from the moment you awake until the moment you rest again? Choose good feeling.

I learned and adapted Louise Hay's quote to this: the way I choose to feel this moment is how I will feel in the next moment; and the next and next. Get it?

If good-feeling is too hard, at least choose better-feeling! That's good enough for me! Wishing you joy on your journey and beauty in your bridge crossings!

Please stay in touch.

With love,

Susan

WITH SUCH GRATITUDE

To Publisher Extraordinaire Sibyl English and to the editors at Sibella Publications International. For finding me on LinkedIn, for offering me the opportunity and for your positive feedback on my writing; without the kind words and encouragement, I would still be just 'wishing I could...'

To my soul-sisters whom I treasure in alphabetical order because there is no measure: Deb — for supporting me 100% always; Laur — for teaching me and always meeting me lovingly where I am; Lela — for being the wind beneath my wings; Nechama — for helping me find my soul and for creating this book, a blessing to me forever.

To the other women in my life: Mom, Mum, Anne, Linda, Rebecca, Sarah; and Robin, Linda S and Lisa P-S — I feel humbled for how much you just love me for who I am, and cheer me on to greater heights. I.LOVE. YOU.

To my husband, thank you for traveling this journey with me. More than ever after all these years, I am yours.

ABOUT THE AUTHOR

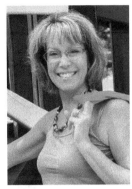

Susan Axelrod, CCP, is the go-to Confidence Coach for Women. Specializing in working with executive women and matriarchs in mid-life who have spent decades doing for others... IT'S YOUR TURN NOW. What does 'my turn' look like? Using co-creative and co-facilitative coaching methods, Susan helps clients uncover the inspired soul within who is looking to live out the second half of life in a self-fulfilling and purposeful way. Susan doesn't give answers or advice. She works with clients to dig into their core, to explore the girl she was and the woman she wants to be for the rest of her life, personally, professionally, spiritually and physically. Using original Confident-Life™ Tools, Susan helps women find the Clarity and Confidence they seek to live out a Best Life. She works with women in transition who declare themselves 'READY!' ...ready to GROW, ready to LIVE now and create a meaningful and lasting legacy. Susan's contagious enthusiasm and deep listening skills spark and motivate clients to get Confident and Thrive!

Susan's Motivational Speaking and Confident-Life Workshops™ are a hit every time! Available for work-teams, book clubs, friend groups, women CEO clubs, nonprofits or any place women gather.

Certified Coach Practitioner, through The Coach Training Academy [accredited by the International Coaching Federation and Certified Coaches Alliance].

CONNECT
WITH SUSAN

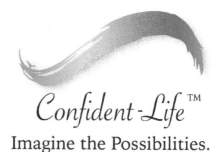

Confident-Life™
Imagine the Possibilities.

Are you ready to live a
more Confident-Life™?

Contact Susan now, you'll be glad you did.

When you call, Susan responds.
Everything is timely, 100% personal and 100% custom.

Please learn about Susan and her work here:
www.whatwillyourlegacybe.com.

CONTACT:
susan@confident-life.com | 518-495-4573

TESTIMONIALS

"My conversation with you helped me so much, in just 20 minutes you really 'got me' and offered a practical reframe. I can't believe how you did that and just seemed to know me right from the start. Your talk gave me something solid and real when I felt like I've been grasping for something for a long time. Your coaching was so helpful and I can't wait to talk to you again. Thank you!"
-Pam Sullivan, Owner of Volution Virtual Services

"I had the opportunity to sit with Susan today at a networking event. It was a brief luncheon conversation, but what she shared with me impacted me to my core. Just from that brief meeting, I am hoping to meet and work with her. She has such an amazing way of communicating and helping you see what you need to for your success. All of this in just a lunch meeting. I can't wait to see what a full session will bring, I recommend Susan to anyone who wants to gain insight."
-Tieece Dixon, Owner of TieBerry Sweets

"Susan, you may not realize it, but our meeting—as brief as it was—really created a lasting impression; think impression like a physical indentation in a surface. The seeds planted that day, especially 'you don't have to be rich to be a philanthropist' resonated on a DNA level. It was more like recognition, like the words settled into a place that already existed for them, if that makes sense. It started a chain reaction and helped create a space where I could really visualize mom's scholarship—when I began to focus on the women it would help. And that gave me the impetus to make it happen by starting to fund the Margaret C. "Peggy" Perkins Memorial Scholarship myself, with the result that in a few weeks, women will be able to apply for the scholarship and the first $1,000 scholarship will be awarded in the Fall."
-Elaine Patrice Perkins, StartUp Grind Albany

CPSIA information can be obtained
at www.ICGtesting.com
Printed in the USA
FFHW012203040519
52234629-57619FF